The Complete Mediterranean Diet Cookbook

Simple and Easy Mediterranean Cookbook, everyone can Cook for an Effortless Weight Loss!

Jose Murphy

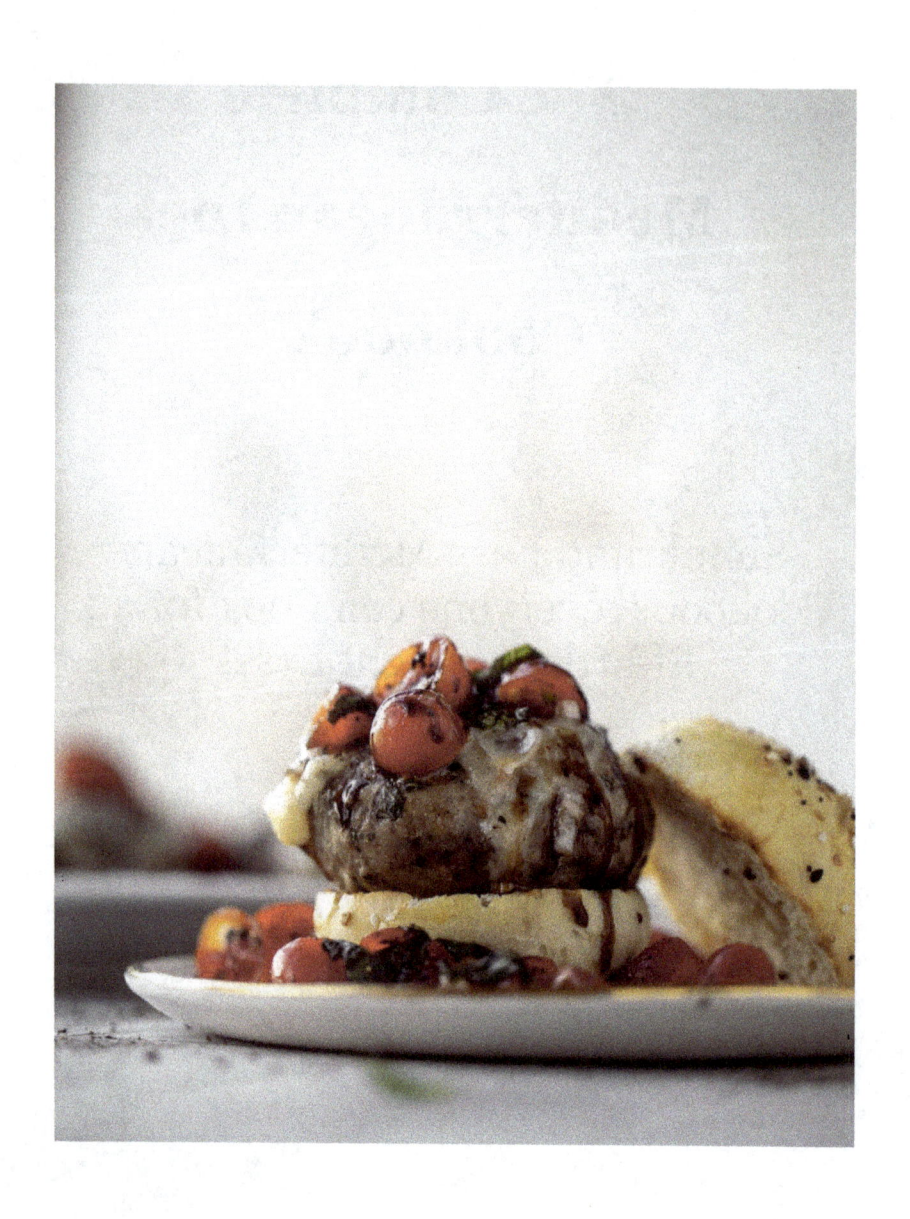

Table of Contents

INTRODUCTION — 7

POULTRY AND MEAT RECIPES — 10

- Chicken Bruschetta Burgers — 10
- Chicken Cacciatore — 12
- Chicken Gyros with Tzatziki Sauce — 14
- Crispy Pesto Chicken — 17
- Beef Stew with Beans and Zucchini — 19
- Greek Beef Kebabs — 23
- Chermoula Roasted Pork Tenderloin — 25
- Lamb Kofta (Spiced Meatballs) — 27
- Chicken and Olives — 30
- Chicken Bake — 32
- Pesto Chicken Mix — 34
- Chicken Wrap — 36
- Chicken and Artichokes — 37
- Chicken Kebabs — 39
- Rosemary Pork Chops — 41
- Pork Chops and Relish — 42
- Pork Chops and Peach Chutney — 45
- — 46
- Glazed Pork Chops — 47
- Pork Chops and Cherries Mix — 49
- Baked Pork Chops — 50

APPETIZER — 51

- Classic Hummus — 51
- Roasted Garlic Hummus — 53
- Red Pepper Hummus — 56
- White Bean Hummus — 58
- Kidney Bean Dip with Cilantro, Cumin, and Lime — 60
- White Bean Dip with Garlic and Herbs — 62
- Black Bean Dip — 65
- Salsa Verde — 67
- Greek Eggplant Dip — 69
- Baba Ghanoush — 71
- Chickpea, Parsley, and Dill Dip — 73

INSTANT POT® SALSA	76
SFOUGATO	78
SKORDALIA	80
PINTO BEAN DIP WITH AVOCADO PICO	82
POWER PODS & HEARTY HAZELNUTS WITH MUSTARD-Y MIX	84
PEPPERY POTATOES	86
TURKEY SPHEROIDS WITH TZATZIKI SAUCE	89
CHEESY CAPRESE SALAD SKEWERS	92
LEAFY LACINATO TUSCAN TREAT	94
GREEK GUACAMOLE HYBRID HUMMUS	95
PORTABLE PACKED PICNIC PIECES	97
PERFECT PIZZA & PASTRY	98
MARGHERITA MEDITERRANEAN MODEL	102
FOWL & FETA FETTUCCINI	104
VERY VEGAN PATRAS PASTA	106
SCRUMPTIOUS SHRIMP PAPPARDELLE PASTA	108
MIXED MUSHROOM PALERMITANI PASTA	111
MEDITERRANEAN MACARONI WITH SEASONED SPINACH	114
FRITTATA FILLED WITH ZESTY ZUCCHINI & TOMATO TOPPINGS	116
CONCLUSION	**118**

© Copyright 2021 by Jose Murphy- All rights reserved.

The following Book is reproduced below with the goal of providing information that is as accurate and reliable as possible. Regardless, purchasing this Book can be seen as consent to the fact that both the publisher and the author of this book are in no way experts on the topics discussed within and that any recommendations or suggestions that are made herein are for entertainment purposes only. Professionals should be consulted as needed prior to undertaking any of the action endorsed herein.

This declaration is deemed fair and valid by both the American Bar Association and the Committee of Publishers Association and is legally binding throughout the United States.

Furthermore, the transmission, duplication, or reproduction of any of the following work including specific information will be considered an illegal act irrespective of if it is done electronically or in print. This extends to creating a secondary or tertiary copy of the work or a recorded copy and is only allowed with the express written consent from the Publisher. All additional right reserved.

The information in the following pages is broadly considered a truthful and accurate account of facts and as such, any inattention, use, or misuse of the information in question by the reader will render any resulting actions solely under their purview. There are no scenarios in which the publisher or the original author of this work can be in any fashion deemed liable for any hardship or damages that may befall them after undertaking information described herein.

Additionally, the information in the following pages is intended only for informational purposes and should thus be thought of as universal. As befitting its nature, it is presented without assurance regarding its prolonged validity or interim quality. Trademarks that are mentioned are done without written consent and can in no way be considered an endorsement from the trademark holder.

INTRODUCTION

The Mediterranean eating regimen is a way of life. It's a method of eating so as to carry on with a full and solid life. When following along these lines of eating you'll get in shape, yet you'll likewise reinforce your heart and give your body all the best possible supplements important to carry on with a long and profitable life. Individuals following the Mediterranean eating regimen have been connected to a lower danger of Alzheimer's malady and malignancy, better generally speaking cardiovascular wellbeing, and an all-inclusive life expectancy. A Mediterranean style eating regimen is joined by a way of life. The way of life has many things that complete the eating routine. It incorporates a lot of exercise, not smoking, drinking in moderation, and having an enthusiasm for your family and life. This is a genuinely effective methodology for keeping up a solid life. The basic premise of this eating routine is that you eat a considerable measure of vegetables, fruits, cereals, nuts, and whole grains. You eat fish or meat scarcely. The omission of meat lessens your hazard of malignancy. You eat some bread. These are a few of the fundamental things that this eating regimen is all about.

The other portion of the Mediterranean eating regimen is the social component. You eat with your loved ones, family, and companions. You profit by the nourishment that you get and you savor your life. You eat inwardly back and center. Your family and companions appreciate it and they likewise figure out how to appreciate it. You meet a few people who are like-minded and you progress toward becoming a family. You get to appreciate your life since you're living it to the most astounding extent conceivable.

You can't take in the Mediterranean eating routine truly unless you be mindful of the exercise, the moderation, and being with the individuals who make it an occurrence to appreciate life. This is for the most part an approach of life. In the event that you need to accomplish the full advantages let this be the best way you choose to live your life. For the most part the general public who are doing it go to the gatherings that are as a rule home based. They have fun, they do things under the sun, and they do issues with their families and clan. They make a decent attempt to live in that sort of setting as opposed to the conventional social environment that a great many people are ordinarily in.

The last piece of the Mediterranean eating regimen is the way of life. One of the things that can be exceptionally harming is the way that you don't chat with your folks sufficiently. You don't get yourself the chance to hear your companions talk about the things that they appreciate, the things that they comprehend, and the things that they be in a position to do for themselves. They appreciate listening to you talk approximately the things that you appreciate, the things that you comprehend, and the things that you can do for yourself. Planning an occasion to get together so you can talk with your companions about your most loved subjects and every one of the underlying intricacies of your life is an essential piece on the way to accomplish the full advantages of the Mediterranean eating routine.

POULTRY AND MEAT RECIPES

Chicken Bruschetta Burgers

Preparation Time: 10 minutes

Cooking Time: 16 minutes

Servings: 2

Ingredients:

- 1 tablespoon olive oil
- 2 garlic cloves, minced
- 3 tablespoons finely minced onion
- 1 teaspoon dried basil
- 3 tablespoons minced sun-dried tomatoes packed in olive oil
- 8 ounces (227 g) ground chicken breast
- ¼ teaspoon salt
- 3 pieces small Mozzarella balls, minced

Directions:

1. Heat the olive oil in a nonstick skillet over medium-high heat. Add the garlic and onion and sauté for 5 minutes until tender. Stir in the basil.
2. Remove from the skillet to a medium bowl.

3. Add the tomatoes, ground chicken, and salt and stir until incorporated. Mix in the Mozzarella balls.
4. Divide the chicken mixture in half and form into two burgers, each about ¾-inch thick.
5. Heat the same skillet over medium-high heat and add the burgers. Cook each side for about 5 to 6 mins. or until they reach an internal temperature of 165°F (74°C).
6. Serve warm.

Nutrition: Calories: 300 Fat: 17.0g Protein: 32.2g Carbs: 6.0g Fiber: 1.1g Sodium: 724mg

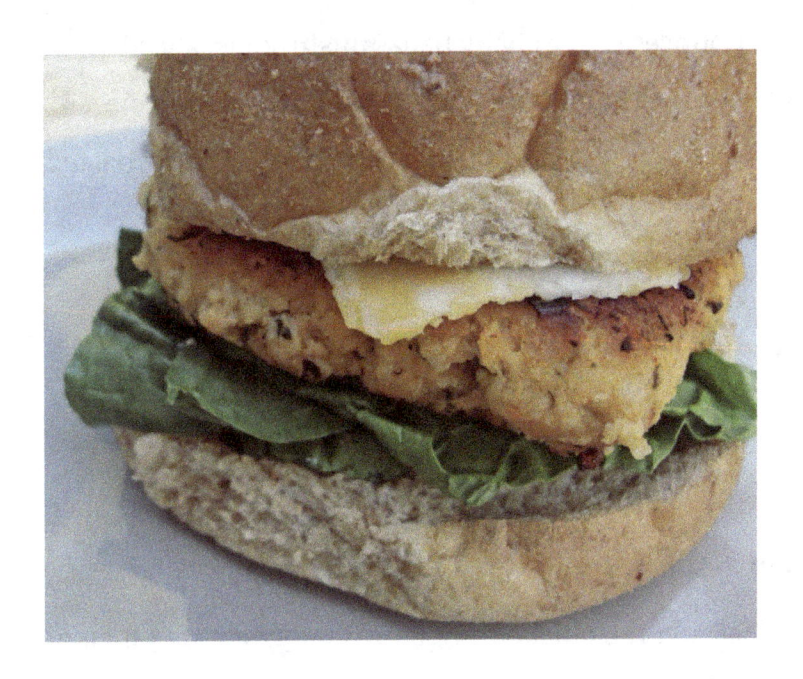

Chicken Cacciatore

Preparation Time: 15 minutes

Cooking Time: 1 hour and 30 minutes

Servings: 2

Ingredients:

- 1½ pounds (680 g) bone-in chicken thighs, skin removed and patted dry
- Salt, to taste
- 2 tablespoons olive oil
- ½ large onion, thinly sliced
- 4 ounces (113 g) baby bella mushrooms, sliced
- 1 red sweet pepper, and then cut into 1-inch pieces
- 1 (15-ounce / 425-g) can crushed fire-roasted tomatoes
- 1 fresh rosemary sprig
- ½ cup dry red wine
- 1 teaspoon Italian herb seasoning
- ½ teaspoon garlic powder
- 3 tablespoons flour

Directions:

1. Season the chicken thighs with a generous pinch of salt.

2. Heat the olive oil in a Dutch oven over medium-high heat. Add the chicken & brown for 5 minutes per side.
3. Add the onion, mushrooms, and sweet pepper to the Dutch oven and sauté for another 5 minutes.
4. Add the tomatoes, rosemary, wine, Italian seasoning, garlic powder, and salt, stirring well.
5. Bring the mixture to a boil, then low the heat to low. Allow to simmer slowly for at least 1 hour, stirring occasionally, or until the chicken is tender and easily pulls away from the bone.
6. Measure out 1 cup of the sauce from the pot and put it into a bowl. Add the flour & whisk well to make a slurry.
7. Now, increase the heat to medium-high and slowly whisk the slurry into the pot. Stir until it comes to a boil and cook until the sauce is thickened.
8. Remove the chicken from the bones and shred it, and add it back to the sauce before serving, if desired.

Nutrition: Calories: 520 Fat: 23.1g Protein: 31.8g Carbs: 37.0g Fiber: 6.0g Sodium: 484mg

Chicken Gyros with Tzatziki Sauce

Preparation Time: 15 minutes

Cooking Time: 10 minutes

Servings: 2

Ingredients:

- 2 tablespoons freshly squeezed lemon juice
- 2 tbsps. olive oil, divided, plus more for oiling the grill
- 1 teaspoon minced fresh oregano
- ½ teaspoon garlic powder
- Salt, to taste
- 8 ounces (227 g) chicken tenders
- 1 small eggplant, cut into 1-inch strips lengthwise
- 1 small zucchini, cut into ½-inch strips lengthwise
- ½ red pepper, seeded and cut in half lengthwise
- ½ English cucumber, peeled and minced
- ¾ cup plain Greek yogurt
- 1 tablespoon minced fresh dill
- 2 (8-inch) pita breads

Directions:

1. Combine the lemon juice, 1 tablespoon of olive oil, oregano, garlic powder, and salt in a medium bowl. Add the chicken and let marinate for 30 minutes.
2. Place the eggplant, zucchini, and red pepper in a large mixing bowl and sprinkle with salt and the remaining 1 tablespoon of olive oil. Toss well to coat. Let the vegetables rest while the chicken is marinating.
3. Make the tzatziki sauce: Combine the cucumber, yogurt, salt, and dill in a medium bowl. Stir well to incorporate and set aside in the refrigerator.
4. When ready, preheat the grill to medium-high heat and oil the grill grates.
5. Drain any liquid from the vegetables and put them on the grill.
6. Remove the chicken tenders from the marinade and put them on the grill.
7. Grill the chicken and vegetables for 3 minutes per side, or until the chicken is no longer pink inside.
8. Remove the chicken and vegetables from the grill and set aside. On the grill, heat the pitas for about 30 seconds, flipping them frequently.
9. Divide the chicken tenders and vegetables between the pitas and top each with ¼ cup of the prepared sauce. Roll the pitas up like a cone and serve.

Nutrition: Calories: 586 Fat: 21.9g Protein: 39.0g Carbs: 62.0g Fiber: 11.8g Sodium: 955mg

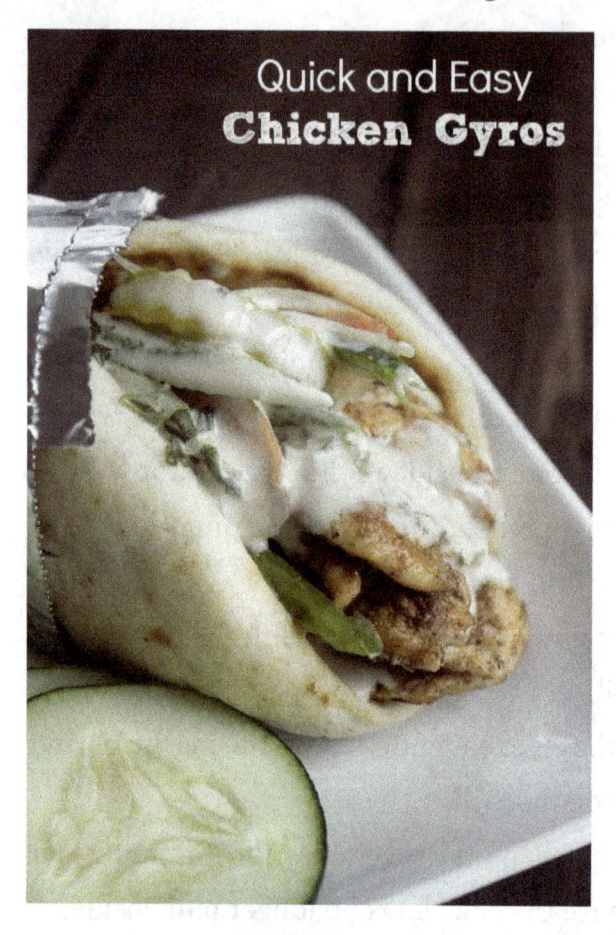

Crispy Pesto Chicken

Preparation Time: 15 minutes

Cooking Time: 50 minutes

Servings: 2

Ingredients:

- 12 ounces (340 g) small red potatoes (3 or 4 potatoes), scrubbed and diced into 1-inch pieces
- 1 tablespoon olive oil
- ½ teaspoon garlic powder
- ¼ teaspoon salt
- 1 (8-ounce / 227-g) boneless, skinless chicken breast
- 3 tablespoons prepared pesto

Directions:

1. Heat your oven to 425°F (220°C). Line a baking sheet with parchment paper.
2. Combine the potatoes, olive oil, garlic powder, and salt in a medium bowl. Toss well to coat.
3. Arrange the potatoes on the parchment paper and roast for 10 minutes. Flip the potatoes and roast for an additional 10 minutes.
4. Meanwhile, put the chicken in the same bowl and toss with the pesto, coating the chicken evenly.

5. Check the potatoes to make sure they are golden brown on the top and bottom. Toss them again and add the chicken breast to the pan.
6. Turn the heat down to 350°F (180°C) and roast the chicken and potatoes for 30 minutes. Check to make sure the chicken reaches an internal temperature of 165°F (74°C) and the potatoes are fork-tender.
7. Let cool for 5 minutes before serving.

Nutrition: Calories: 378 Fat: 16.0g Protein: 29.8g Carbs: 30.1g Fiber: 4.0g Sodium: 425mg

Beef Stew with Beans and Zucchini

Preparation Time: 20 minutes

Cooking Time: 6 to 8 hours

Servings: 2

Ingredients:

- 1 (15-ounce / 425-g) can diced or crushed tomatoes with basil
- 1 teaspoon beef base
- 2 tablespoons olive oil, divided
- 8 ounces (227 g) baby bella (cremini) mushrooms, quartered
- 2 garlic cloves, minced
- ½ large onion, diced
- 1 pound (454 g) cubed beef stew meat
- 3 tablespoons flour
- ¼ teaspoon salt
- Pinch freshly ground black pepper
- ¾ cup dry red wine
- ¼ cup minced brined olives
- 1 fresh rosemary sprig
- 1 (15-ounce / 425-g) can white cannellini beans, drained and rinsed

- One medium zucchini, cut in half lengthwise and then cut into 1-inch pieces.

Directions:

1. Place the tomatoes into a slow cooker and set it to low heat. Add the beef base and stir to incorporate.
2. Heat 1 tablespoon of olive oil in a large sauté pan over medium heat.
3. Add the mushrooms and onion and sauté for 10 minutes, stirring occasionally, or until they're golden.
4. Add the garlic and cook for 30 seconds more. Transfer the vegetables to the slow cooker.
5. In a plastic food storage bag, combine the stew meat with the flour, salt, and pepper. Seal the bag & shake well to combine.
6. Heat the remaining 1 tablespoon of olive oil in the sauté pan over high heat.
7. Add the floured meat and sear to get a crust on the outside edges. Deglaze the pan by adding about half of the red wine and scraping up any browned bits on the bottom. Stir so the wine thickens a bit and transfer to the slow cooker along with any remaining wine.

8. Stir the stew to incorporate the ingredients. Stir in the olives and rosemary, cover, and cook for 6 to 8 hours on Low.
9. About 30 minutes before the stew is finished, add the beans and zucchini to let them warm through. Serve warm.

Nutrition: Calories: 389 Fat: 15.1g Protein: 30.8g Carbs: 25.0g Fiber: 8.0g Sodium: 582mg

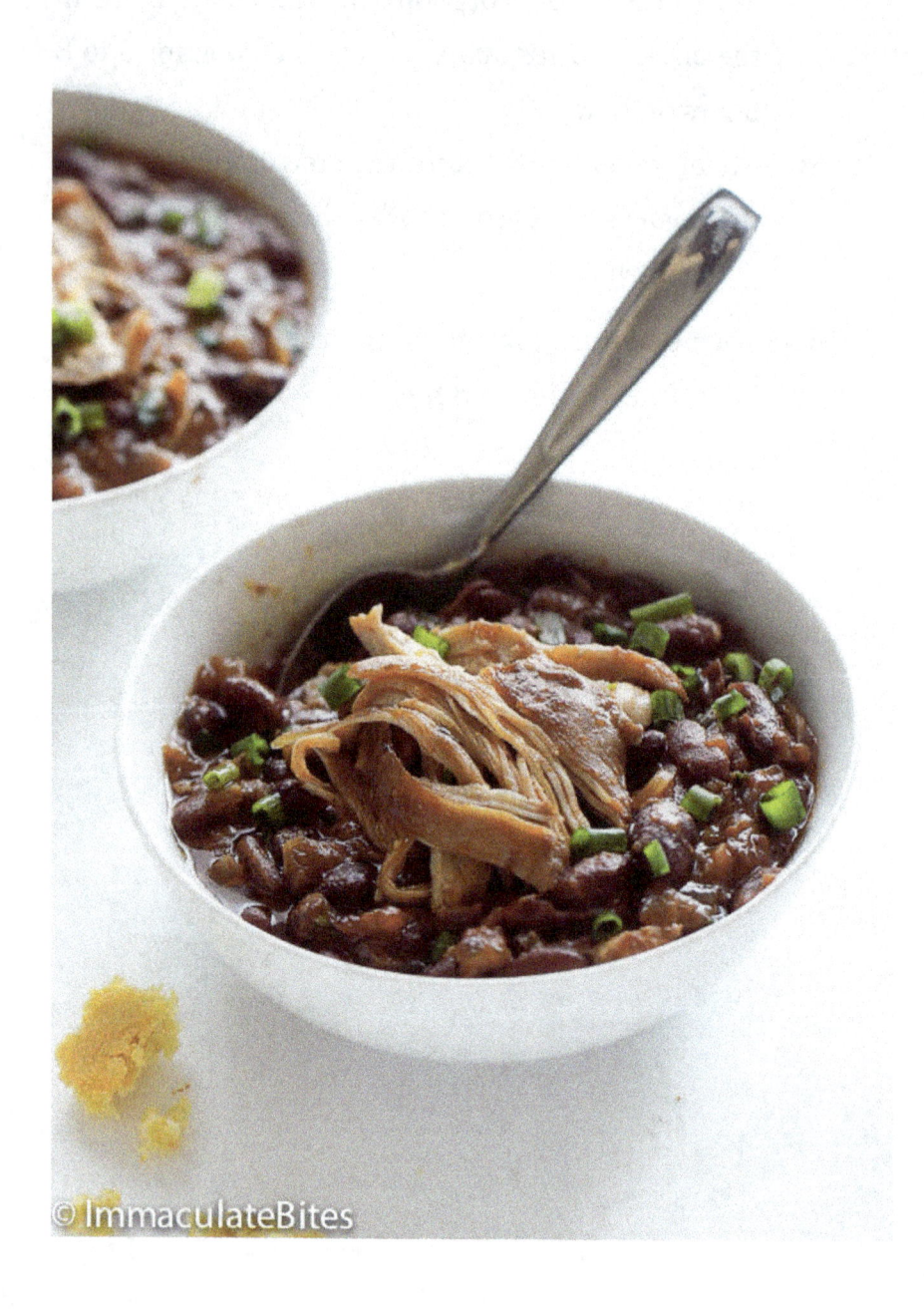

Greek Beef Kebabs

Preparation Time: 15 minutes

Cooking Time: 20 minutes

Servings: 2

Ingredients:

- 6 ounces (170 g) beef sirloin tip, trimmed of Fat and cut into 2-inch pieces
- 3 cups of any mixture of vegetables: mushrooms, summer squash, zucchini, onions, red peppers, cherry tomatoes
- ½ cup olive oil
- ¼ cup freshly squeezed lemon juice
- 2 tablespoons balsamic vinegar
- 2 teaspoons dried oregano
- 1 teaspoon garlic powder
- 1 teaspoon salt
- 1 teaspoon minced fresh rosemary
- Cooking spray

Directions:

1. Put the beef in a plastic freezer bag.
2. Slice the vegetables into similar-size pieces and put them in a second freezer bag.

3. Make the marinade: Mix the olive oil, lemon juice, balsamic vinegar, oregano, garlic powder, salt, and rosemary in a measuring cup. Whisk well to combine. Pour half of marinade over the beef, and the other half over the vegetables.
4. Put the beef and vegetables in the refrigerator to marinate for 4 hours.
5. When ready, preheat the grill to medium-high heat and spray the grill grates with cooking spray.
6. Thread the meat onto skewers and the vegetables onto separate skewers.
7. Grill the meat for 3 mins per side. They should only take 10 to 12 minutes to cook, depending on the thickness of the meat.
8. Grill the vegetables for about 3 minutes per side, or until they have grill marks and are softened.
9. Serve hot.

Nutrition: Calories: 284 Fat: 18.2g Protein: 21.0g Carbs: 9.0g Fiber: 3.9g Sodium: 122mg

Chermoula Roasted Pork Tenderloin

Preparation Time: 15 minutes

Cooking Time: 20 minutes

Servings: 2

Ingredients:

- ½ cup fresh cilantro
- ½ cup fresh parsley
- 6 small garlic cloves
- 3 tablespoons olive oil, divided
- 3 tablespoons freshly squeezed lemon juice
- 2 teaspoons cumin
- 1 teaspoon smoked paprika
- ½ teaspoon salt, divided
- Pinch freshly ground black pepper
- 1 (8-ounce / 227-g) pork tenderloin

Directions:

1. Heat your oven to 425°F (220°C).
2. In a food processor, combine the cilantro, parsley, garlic, 2 tablespoons of olive oil, lemon juice, cumin, paprika, and ¼ teaspoon of salt. Pulse 15 to 20 times, or until the mixture is fairly smooth. Scrape the sides down as needed to incorporate all the

ingredients. Transfer the sauce into a small bowl & set aside.

3. Season the pork tenderloin on all sides with the remaining ¼ teaspoon of salt and a generous pinch of black pepper.
4. Heat the remaining 1 tablespoon of olive oil in a sauté pan.
5. Sear the pork for 3 minutes, turning often, until golden brown on all sides.
6. Transfer the pork into a baking dish & roast in the preheated oven for 15 minutes, or until the internal temperature registers 145°F (63°C).
7. Cool for 5 minutes before serving.

Nutrition: Calories: 169 Fat: 13.1g Protein: 11.0g Carbs: 2.9g Fiber: 1.0g Sodium: 332mg

Lamb Kofta (Spiced Meatballs)

Preparation Time: 15 minutes

Cooking Time: 30 minutes

Servings: 2

Ingredients:

- ¼ cup walnuts
- 1 garlic clove
- ½ small onion
- 1 roasted piquillo pepper
- 2 tablespoons fresh mint
- 2 tablespoons fresh parsley
- ¼ teaspoon cumin
- ¼ teaspoon allspice
- ¼ teaspoon salt
- Pinch cayenne pepper
- 8 ounces (227 g) lean ground lamb

Directions:

1. Heat your oven to 350°F (180°C). Line a baking sheet with aluminum foil.
2. In a food processor, combine the walnuts, garlic, onion, roasted pepper, mint, parsley, cumin,

allspice, salt, and cayenne pepper. Pulse about 10 times to combine everything.

3. Transfer the spice mixture to a large bowl and add the ground lamb. With your hands or a spatula, mix the spices into the lamb.
4. Roll the lamb into 1½-inch balls (about the size of golf balls).
5. Arrange the meatballs on the prepared baking sheet and bake for 30 minutes, or until cooked to an internal temperature of 165°F (74°C).
6. Serve warm.

Nutrition: Calories: 409 Fat: 22.9g Protein: 22.0g Carbs: 7.1g Fiber: 3.0g Sodium: 428mg

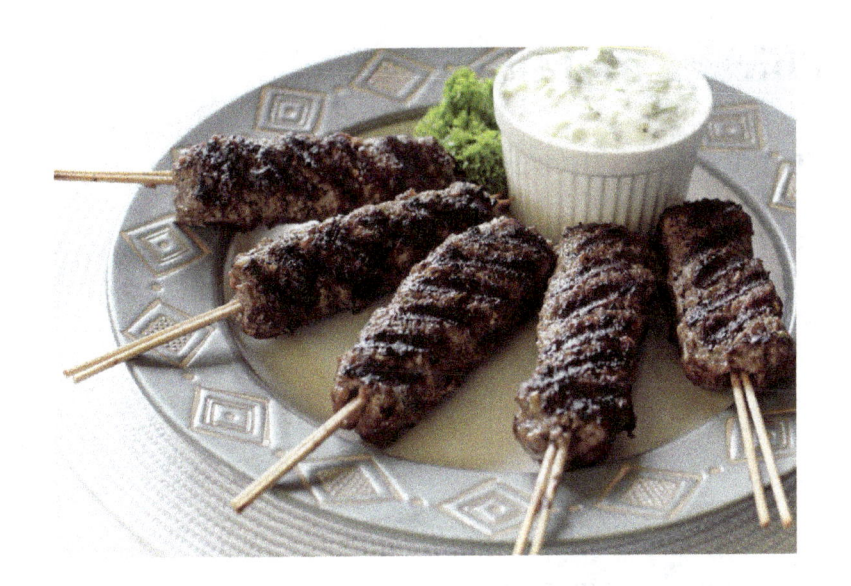

Chicken and Olives

Preparation Time: 10 minutes

Cooking Time: 15 minutes

Servings: 4

Ingredients:

- 4 chicken breasts, skinless and boneless
- 2 tablespoons garlic, minced
- 1 tablespoon oregano, dried
- Salt and black pepper to the taste
- 2 tablespoons olive oil
- ½ cup chicken stock
- Juice of 1 lemon
- 1 cup red onion, chopped
- 1 and ½ cups tomatoes, cubed
- ¼ cup green olives, pitted and sliced
- A handful parsley, chopped

Directions:

1. Heat up a pan w/ the oil over medium-high heat, add the chicken, garlic, salt and pepper and brown for 2 minutes on each side.

2. Add the rest of the ingredients, toss, bring the mix to a simmer and cook over medium heat for 13 minutes.
3. Divide the mix between plates and serve.

Nutrition: Calories 135, Fat 5.8, Fiber 3.4, Carbs 12.1, Protein 9.6

Chicken Bake

Preparation Time: 10 minutes

Cooking Time: 30 minutes

Servings: 4

Ingredients:

- 1 and ½ pounds chicken thighs, skinless, boneless and cubed
- 2 garlic cloves, minced
- 1 tablespoon oregano, chopped
- 2 tablespoons olive oil
- 1 tablespoon red wine vinegar
- ½ cup canned artichokes, drained and chopped
- 1 red onion, sliced
- 1 pound whole wheat fusili pasta, cooked
- ½ cup canned white beans, drained and rinsed
- ½ cup parsley, chopped
- 1 cup mozzarella, shredded
- Salt and black pepper to the taste

Directions:

1. Heat up a pan with half of the oil over medium-high heat, add the meat and brown for 5 minutes.

2. Grease a baking pan with the rest of the oil, add the browned chicken, and the rest of the ingredients except the pasta and the mozzarella.
3. Spread the pasta all over and toss gently.
4. Now, sprinkle the mozzarella on top and bake at 425 degrees F for 25 minutes.
5. Divide the bake between plates and serve.

Nutrition: Calories 195, Fat 5.8, Fiber 3.4, Carbs 12.1, Protein 11.6

Pesto Chicken Mix

Preparation Time: 10 minutes

Cooking Time: 40 minutes

Servings: 4

Ingredients:

- 4 chicken breast halves, skinless and boneless
- 3 tomatoes, cubed
- 1 cup mozzarella, shredded
- ½ cup basil pesto
- A pinch of salt and black pepper
- Cooking spray

Directions:

1. Grease a baking dish lined with parchment paper with the cooking spray.
2. In a bowl, mix the chicken with salt, pepper and the pesto and rub well.
3. Place the chicken on the baking sheet, top with tomatoes and shredded mozzarella and bake at 400 degrees F for 40 mins.
4. Divide the mix between plates & serve with a side salad.

Nutrition: Calories 341, Fat 20, Fiber 1, Carbs 4, Protein 32

Chicken Wrap

Preparation Time: 10 minutes

Cooking Time: 0 minutes

Servings: 2

Ingredients:

- 2 whole wheat tortilla flatbreads
- 6 chicken breast slices, skinless, boneless, cooked and shredded
- A handful baby spinach
- 2 provolone cheese slices
- 4 tomato slices
- 10 kalamata olives, pitted and sliced
- 1 red onion, sliced
- 2 tablespoons roasted peppers, chopped

Directions:

1. Arrange the tortillas on a working surface, and divide the chicken and the other ingredients on each.
2. Roll the tortillas and serve them right away.

Nutrition: Calories 190, Fat 6.8, Fiber 3.5, Carbs 15.1, Protein 6.6

Chicken and Artichokes

Preparation Time: 10 minutes

Cooking Time: 20 minutes

Servings: 4

Ingredients:

- 2 pounds chicken breast, skinless, boneless and sliced
- A pinch of salt and black pepper
- 4 tablespoons olive oil
- 8 ounces canned roasted artichoke hearts, drained
- 6 ounces sun-dried tomatoes, chopped
- 3 tablespoons capers, drained
- 2 tablespoons lemon juice

Directions:

1. Heat up a pan with half of the oil over medium-high heat, add the artichokes and the other ingredients except the chicken, stir and sauté for 10 minutes.
2. Transfer the mix to a bowl, heat up the pan again with the rest of the oil over medium-high heat, add the meat and cook for 4 minutes on each side.

3. Return the veggie mix to the pan, toss, cook everything for 2-3 minutes more, divide between plates and serve.

Nutrition: Calories 552, Fat 28, Fiber 6, Carbs 33, Protein 43

Chicken Kebabs

Preparation Time: 30 minutes

Cooking Time: 20 minutes

Servings: 4

Ingredients:

- 2 chicken breasts, skinless, boneless and cubed
- 1 red bell pepper, cut into squares
- 1 red onion, roughly cut into squares
- 2 teaspoons sweet paprika
- 1 teaspoon nutmeg, ground
- 1 teaspoon Italian seasoning
- ¼ teaspoon smoked paprika
- A pinch of salt and black pepper
- ¼ teaspoon cardamom, ground
- Juice of 1 lemon
- 3 garlic cloves, minced
- ½ cup olive oil

Directions:

1. Combine the chicken with the onion, the bell pepper and the other ingredients, toss well, cover the bowl and keep in the fridge for 30 minutes.

2. Assemble skewers with chicken, peppers and the onions, place them on your preheated grill and cook over medium heat for 8 minutes on each side.
3. Divide the kebabs between plates and serve with a side salad.

Nutrition: Calories 262, Fat 14, Fiber 2, Carbs 14, Protein 20

Rosemary Pork Chops

Preparation Time: 10 minutes

Cooking Time: 35 minutes

Servings: 4

Ingredients:

- 4 pork loin chops, boneless
- Salt and black pepper to the taste
- 4 garlic cloves, minced
- 1 tablespoon rosemary, chopped
- 1 tablespoon olive oil

Directions:

1. In a roasting pan, combine the pork chops with the rest of the ingredients, toss, and bake at 425 degrees F for 10 min.
2. Low the heat to 350 degrees F and cook the chops for 25 minutes more.
3. Divide the chops between plates and serve with a side salad.

Nutrition: Calories 161, Fat 5, Fiber 1, Carbs 1, Protein 25

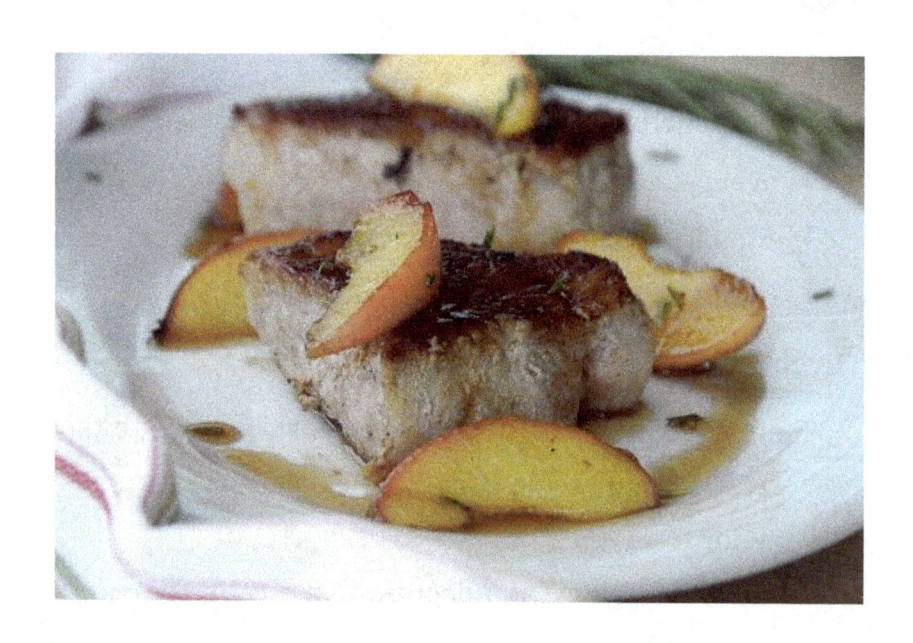

Pork Chops and Relish

Preparation Time: 15 minutes

Cooking Time: 14 minutes

Servings: 6

Ingredients:

- 6 pork chops, boneless
- 7 ounces marinated artichoke hearts, chopped and their liquid reserved
- A pinch of salt and black pepper
- 1 teaspoon hot pepper sauce
- 1 and ½ cups tomatoes, cubed
- 1 jalapeno pepper, chopped
- ½ cup roasted bell peppers, chopped
- ½ cup black olives, pitted and sliced

Directions:

1. In a bowl, mix the chops with the pepper sauce, reserved liquid from the artichokes, cover and keep in the fridge for 15 minutes.
2. Heat up a grill over medium-high heat, add the pork chops and cook for 7 minutes on each side.

3. In a bowl, combine the artichokes with the peppers and the remaining ingredients, toss, divide on top of the chops and serve.

Nutrition: Calories 215, Fat 6, Fiber 1, Carbs 6, Protein 35

Pork Chops and Peach Chutney

Preparation Time: 10 minutes

Cooking Time: 30 minutes

Servings: 4

Ingredients:

- 4 pork loin chops, boneless
- Salt and black pepper to the taste
- ½ teaspoon garlic powder
- ¼ teaspoon cumin, ground
- ½ teaspoon sage, dried
- Cooking spray
- 1 teaspoon chili powder
- 1 teaspoon oregano, dried

For the chutney:

- ¼ cup shallot, minced
- 1 teaspoon olive oil
- 2 cups peaches, peeled and chopped
- ½ cup red sweet pepper, chopped
- 2 tablespoons jalapeno chili pepper, minced
- 1 tablespoon balsamic vinegar
- ½ teaspoon cinnamon powder
- 2 tablespoons cilantro, chopped

Directions:

1. Heat up a pan w/ the olive oil over medium heat, add the shallot and sauté for 5 minutes.
2. Add the sweet pepper, peaches, chili pepper, vinegar, cinnamon and the cilantro, stir, simmer for 10 minutes and take off the heat.
3. Meanwhile, in a bowl, combine the pork chops with cooking spray, salt, pepper, garlic powder, cumin, sage, oregano and chili powder and rub well.
4. Heat up your grill over medium-high heat, add pork chops, cook for 6-7 minutes on each side, divide between plates and serve with the chutney on top.

Nutrition: Calories 297, Fat 10, Fiber 2, Carbs 13, Protein 38

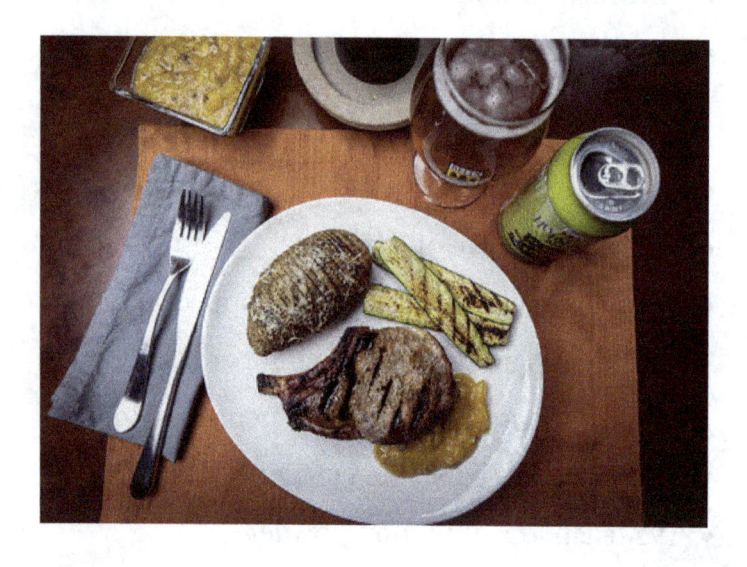

Glazed Pork Chops

Preparation Time: 10 minutes

Cooking Time: 20 minutes

Servings: 4

Ingredients:

- ¼ cup apricot preserves
- 4 pork chops, boneless
- 1 tablespoon thyme, chopped
- ½ teaspoon cinnamon powder
- 2 tablespoons olive oil

Directions:

1. Heat up a pan w/ the oil over medium-high heat, add the apricot preserves and cinnamon, whisk, bring to a simmer, cook for 10 minutes and take off the heat.
2. Heat up your grill over medium-high heat, brush the pork chops with some of the apricot glaze, place them on the grill and cook for 10 minutes.
3. Flip the chops, brush them with more apricot glaze, cook for 10 minutes more and divide between plates.
4. Sprinkle the thyme on top and serve.

Nutrition: Calories 225, Fat 11, Fiber 0, Carbs 6, Protein 23

Pork Chops and Cherries Mix

Preparation Time: 10 minutes

Cooking Time: 12 minutes

Servings: 4

Ingredients:

- 4 pork chops, boneless
- Salt and black pepper to the taste
- ½ cup cranberry juice
- 1 and ½ teaspoons spicy mustard
- ½ cup dark cherries, pitted and halved
- Cooking spray

Directions:

1. Heat up a pan greased with the cooking spray over medium-high heat, add the pork chops, cook them for 5 minutes on each side and divide between plates.
2. Heat up the same pan over medium heat, add the cranberry juice and the rest of the ingredients, whisk, bring to a simmer, cook for 2 minutes, drizzle over the pork chops and serve.

Nutrition: Calories 262, Fat 8, Fiber 1, Carbs 16, Protein 30

Baked Pork Chops

Preparation Time: 10 minutes

Cooking Time: 30 minutes

Servings: 4

Ingredients:

- 4 pork loin chops, boneless
- A pinch of salt and black pepper
- 1 tablespoon sweet paprika
- 2 tablespoons Dijon mustard
- Cooking spray

Directions:

1. In a bowl, mix the pork chops with salt, pepper, paprika and the mustard and rub well.
2. Grease a baking sheet with cooking spray, add the pork chops, cover with tin foil, introduce in the oven and bake at 400 degrees F for 30 minutes.
3. Divide the pork chops between plates and serve with a side salad.

Nutrition: Calories 167, Fat 5, Fiber 0, Carbs 2, Protein 25

APPETIZER

Classic Hummus

Preparation Time: 8 minutes

Cooking Time: 30 minutes

Serving: 6

Size/ Portion: 2 tablespoons

Ingredient:

- 1 cup dried chickpeas
- 4 cups water
- 1 tablespoon plus ¼ cup extra-virgin olive oil
- 1/3 cup tahini
- 1½ teaspoons ground cumin
- ¾ teaspoon salt
- ½ teaspoon ground black pepper
- ½ teaspoon ground coriander
- 1/3 cup lemon juice

- 1 teaspoon minced garlic

Direction:

1. Position chickpeas, water, and 1 tablespoon oil in the Instant Pot®. Close, select steam release to Sealing, click Manual, and time to 30 minutes.

2. When the timer rings, quick-release the pressure and open lid. Press the Cancel button and open lid. Drain, reserving the cooking liquid.

3. Blend chickpeas, remaining ¼ cup oil, tahini, cumin, salt, pepper, coriander, lemon juice, and garlic in a food processor. Serve.

Nutrition: 152 Calories 12g Fat 4g Protein

Roasted Garlic Hummus

Preparation Time: 9 minutes

Cooking Time: 33 minutes

Serving: 4

Size/ Portion: 2 tablespoons

Ingredients:

- 1 cup dried chickpeas
- 4 cups water
- 1 tablespoon plus ¼ cup extra-virgin olive oil, divided
- 1/3 cup tahini
- 1 teaspoon ground cumin
- ½ teaspoon onion powder
- ¾ teaspoon salt
- ½ teaspoon ground black pepper
- 1/3 cup lemon juice
- 3 tablespoons mashed roasted garlic

- 2 tablespoons chopped fresh parsley

Direction:

1. Situate chickpeas, water, and 1 tablespoon oil in the Instant Pot®. Cover, press steam release to Sealing, set Manual button, and time to 30 minutes.

2. When the timer beeps, quick-release the pressure. Select Cancel button and open. Strain, reserving the cooking liquid.

3. Place chickpeas, remaining ¼ cup oil, tahini, cumin, onion powder, salt, pepper, lemon juice, and roasted garlic in a food processor and process until creamy. Top with parsley. Serve at room temperature.

Nutrition: 104 Calories 6g Fat 4g Protein

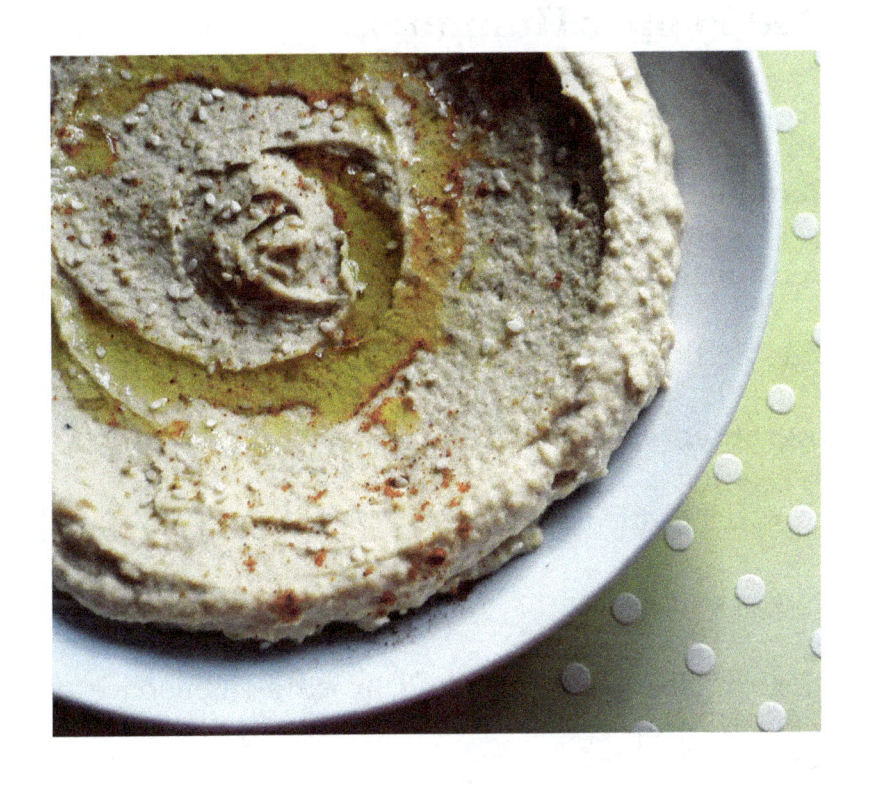

Red Pepper Hummus

Preparation Time: 7 minutes

Cooking Time: 34 minutes

Serving: 4

Size/ Portion: 2 tablespoons

Ingredients:

- 1 cup dried chickpeas
- 4 cups water
- 1 tablespoon plus ¼ cup extra-virgin olive oil, divided
- ½ cup chopped roasted red pepper, divided
- 1/3 cup tahini
- 1 teaspoon ground cumin
- ¾ teaspoon salt
- ½ teaspoon ground black pepper
- ¼ teaspoon smoked paprika
- 1/3 cup lemon juice

- ½ teaspoon minced garlic

Direction:

1. Put chickpeas, water, and 1 tablespoon oil in the Instant Pot®. Seal, put steam release to Sealing, select Manual and time to 30 minutes.

2. When the timer rings, quick-release the pressure. Click Cancel button and open it. Drain, set aside the cooking liquid.

3. Process chickpeas, 1/3 cup roasted red pepper, remaining ¼ cup oil, tahini, cumin, salt, black pepper, paprika, lemon juice, and garlic using food processor. Serve, garnished with reserved roasted red pepper on top.

Nutrition: 96 Calories 8g Fat 2g Protein

White Bean Hummus

Preparation Time: 11 minutes

Cooking Time: 40 minutes

Serving: 12

Size/ Portion: 4 tablespoons

Ingredients:

- 2/3 cup dried white beans
- 3 cloves garlic, peeled and crushed
- ¼ cup olive oil
- 1 tablespoon lemon juice
- ½ teaspoon salt

Direction

1. Place beans and garlic in the Instant Pot® and stir well. Add enough cold water to cover ingredients. Cover, set steam release to Sealing, select Manual button, and time to 30 minutes.

2. Once the timer stops, release pressure for 20 minutes. Select Cancel and open lid. Use a fork to

check that beans are tender. Drain off excess water and transfer beans to a food processor.

3. Add oil, lemon juice, and salt to the processor and pulse until mixture is smooth with some small chunks. Pour into container and refrigerate for at least 4 hours. Serve cold or at room temperature.

Nutrition: 57 Calories 5g Fat 1g Protein

Kidney Bean Dip with Cilantro, Cumin, and Lime

Preparation Time: 13 minutes

Cooking Time: 51 minutes

Serving: 16

Size/ Portion: 2 tablespoons

Ingredients:

- 1 cup dried kidney beans
- 4 cups water
- 3 cloves garlic
- ¼ cup cilantro
- ¼ cup extra-virgin olive oil
- 1 tablespoon lime juice
- 2 teaspoons grated lime zest
- 1 teaspoon ground cumin
- ½ teaspoon salt

Direction

1. Place beans, water, garlic, and 2 tablespoons cilantro in the Instant Pot®. Close the lid, select steam release to Sealing, click Bean button, and cook for 30 minutes.

2. When the timer alarms, let pressure release naturally, about 20 minutes. Press the Cancel button, open lid, and check that beans are tender. Drain off extra water and transfer beans to a medium bowl. Gently mash beans with potato masher. Add oil, lime juice, lime zest, cumin, salt, and remaining 2 tablespoons cilantro and stir to combine. Serve warm or at room temperature.

Nutrition: 65 Calories 3g Fat 2g Protein

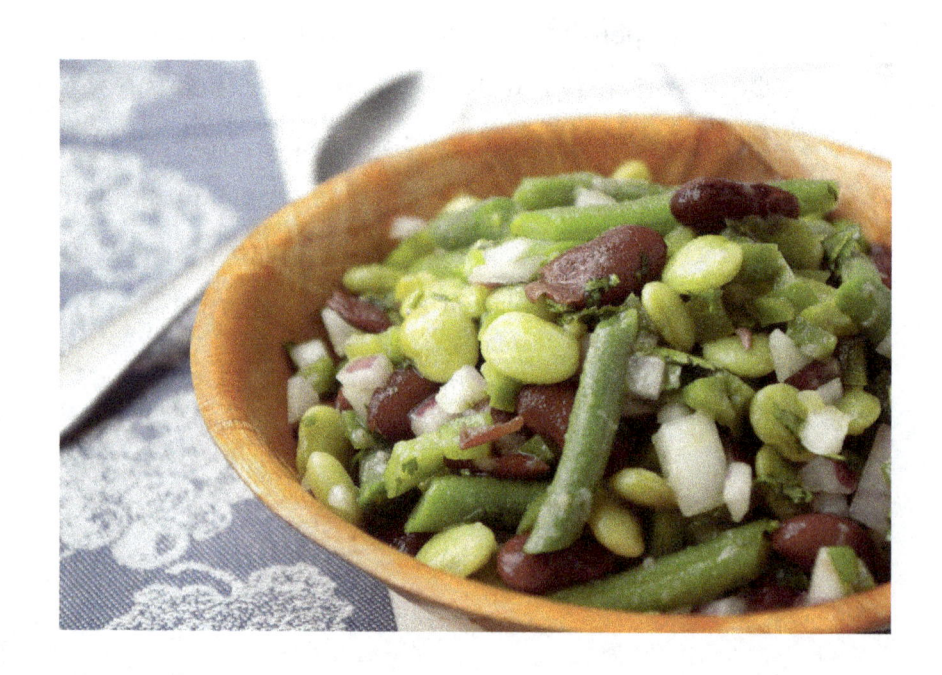

White Bean Dip with Garlic and Herbs

Preparation Time: 10 minutes

Cooking Time: 48 minutes

Serving: 16

Size/ Portion: 2 tablespoons

Ingredients:

- 1 cup dried white beans
- 3 cloves garlic
- 8 cups water
- ¼ cup extra-virgin olive oil
- ¼ cup chopped fresh flat-leaf parsley
- 1 tablespoon fresh oregano
- 1 tablespoon d fresh tarragon
- 1 teaspoon fresh thyme leaves
- 1 teaspoon lemon zest
- ¼ teaspoon salt

- ¼ teaspoon black pepper

Direction

1. Place beans and garlic in the Instant Pot® and stir well. Add water, close lid, put steam release to Sealing, press the Manual, and adjust time to 30 minutes.

2. When the timer beeps, release naturally, about 20 minutes. Open and check if beans are soft. Press the Cancel button, drain off excess water, and transfer beans and garlic to a food processor with olive oil. Add parsley, oregano, tarragon, thyme, lemon zest, salt, and pepper, and pulse 3–5 times to mix. Chill for 4 hours or overnight. Serve cold or at room temperature.

Nutrition: 47 Calories 3g Fat 1g Protein

Black Bean Dip

Preparation Time: 14 minutes

Cooking Time: 53 minutes

Serving: 16

Size/ Portion: 2 tablespoons

Ingredients:

- 1 tablespoon olive oil
- 2 slices bacon
- 1 small onion,
- 3 cloves garlic
- 1 cup low-sodium chicken broth
- 1 cup dried black beans
- 1 (14.5-ounce) can diced tomatoes
- 1 small jalapeño pepper
- 1 teaspoon ground cumin
- ½ teaspoon smoked paprika
- 1 tablespoon lime juice

- ½ teaspoon dried oregano
- ¼ cup minced fresh cilantro
- ¼ teaspoon sea salt

Direction:

1. Press the Sauté button on the Instant Pot® and heat oil. Add bacon and onion. Cook for 5 minutes. Cook garlic for 30 seconds. Add broth and scrape any browned bits from bottom of pot. Add beans, tomatoes, jalapeño, cumin, paprika, lime juice, oregano, cilantro, and salt. Press the Cancel button.

2. Close lid, let steam release to Sealing, set Bean button, and default time of 30 minutes. When the timer rings, let pressure release naturally for 10 minutes. Press the Cancel button and open lid.

3. Use an immersion blender blend the ingredients. Serve warm.

Nutrition: 60 Calories 2g Fat 3g Protein

Salsa Verde

Preparation Time: 9 minutes

Cooking Time: 21 minutes

Serving: 8

Size/ Portion: 2 tablespoons

Ingredients:

- 1-pound tomatillos
- 2 small jalapeño peppers
- 1 small onion
- ½ cup chopped fresh cilantro
- 1 teaspoon ground coriander
- 1 teaspoon sea salt
- 1½ cups water

Direction:

1. Cut tomatillos in half and place in the Instant Pot®. Add enough water to cover.

2. Close lids, set steam release to Sealing, press the Manual button, and set time to 2 minutes. Once

timer beeps, release pressure naturally, for 20 minutes. Press the Cancel and open lid.

3. Drain off excess water and transfer tomatillos to a food processor or blender, and add jalapeños, onion, cilantro, coriander, salt, and water. Pulse until well combined, about 20 pulses.

4. Wrap and cool for 2 hours before serving.

Nutrition: 27 Calories 1g Fat 1g Protein

Greek Eggplant Dip

Preparation Time: 16 minutes

Cooking Time: 3 minutes

Serving: 8

Size/ Portion: 2 tablespoons

Ingredients:

- 1 cup water
- 1 large eggplant
- 1 clove garlic
- ½ teaspoon salt
- 1 tablespoon red wine vinegar
- ½ cup extra-virgin olive oil
- 2 tablespoons minced fresh parsley

Direction

1. Add water to the Instant Pot®, add the rack to the pot, and place the steamer basket on the rack.
2. Place eggplant in steamer basket. Close, set steam release to Sealing, turn on Manual button, and set

time to 3 minutes. When the timer stops, quick-release the pressure. Click Cancel button and open.

3. Situate eggplant to a food processor and add garlic, salt, and vinegar. Pulse until smooth, about 20 pulses.

4. Slowly add oil to the eggplant mixture while the food processor runs continuously until oil is completely incorporated. Stir in parsley. Serve at room temperature.

Nutrition: 134 Calories 14g Fat 1g Protein

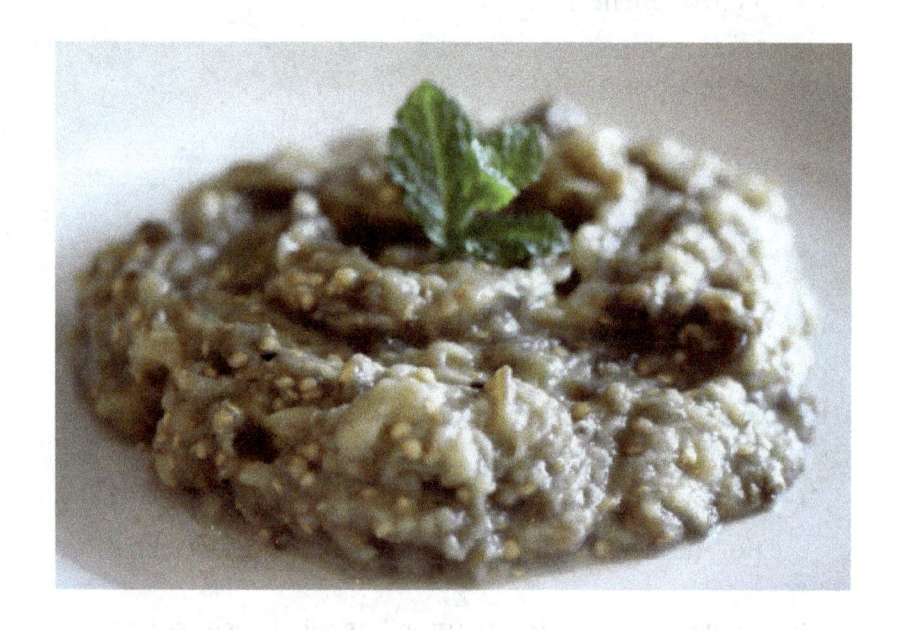

Baba Ghanoush

Preparation Time: 9 minutes

Cooking Time: 11 minutes

Serving: 8

Size/ Portion: 3 tablespoons

Ingredients:

- 2 tablespoons extra-virgin olive oil
- 1 large eggplant
- 3 cloves garlic
- ½ cup water
- 3 tablespoons fresh flat-leaf parsley
- ½ teaspoon salt
- ¼ teaspoon smoked paprika
- 2 tablespoons lemon juice
- 2 tablespoons tahini

Direction

1. Press the Sauté button on the Instant Pot® and add 1 tablespoon oil. Add eggplant and cook until it begins to soften, about 5 minutes. Add garlic and cook 30 seconds.

2. Add water and close lid, click steam release to Sealing, select Manual, and time to 6 minutes. Once the timer rings, quick-release the pressure. Select Cancel and open lid.

3. Strain cooked eggplant and garlic and add to a food processor or blender along with parsley, salt, smoked paprika, lemon juice, and tahini. Add remaining 1 tablespoon oil and process. Serve warm or at room temperature.

Nutrition: 79 Calories 6g Fat 2g Protein

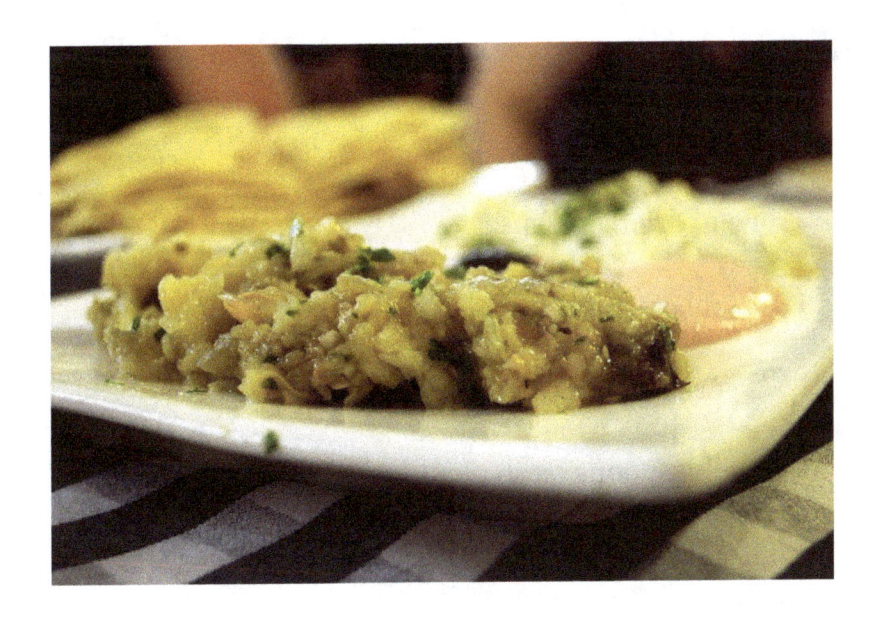

Chickpea, Parsley, and Dill Dip

Preparation Time: 11 minutes

Cooking Time: 22 minutes

Serving: 6

Size/ Portion: 2 tablespoons

Ingredients:

- 8 cups water
- 1 cup dried chickpeas
- 3 tablespoons olive oil
- 2 garlic cloves
- 2 tablespoons fresh parsley
- 2 tablespoons fresh dill
- 1 tablespoon lemon juice
- ¼ teaspoon salt

Direction

1. Add 4 cups water and chickpeas to the Instant Pot®. Cover, place steam release to Sealing. Set Manual,

and time to 1 minute. When the timer beeps, quick-release the pressure until the float valve drops, press the Cancel button, and open lid.

2. Drain water, rinse chickpeas, and return to pot with 4 cups fresh water. Set aside to soak for 1 hour.

3. Add 1 tablespoon oil to pot. Close, adjust steam release to Sealing, click Manual, and the time to 20 minutes. When alarm beeps, let pressure release for 20 minutes. Click the Cancel, open and drain chickpeas.

4. Place chickpeas to a food processor or blender, and add garlic, parsley, dill, lemon juice, and remaining 2 tablespoons water. Blend for about 30 seconds.

5. With the processor or blender lid still in place, slowly add remaining 2 tablespoons oil while still blending, then add salt. Serve warm or at room temperature.

Nutrition: 76 Calories 4g Fat 2g Protein

Instant Pot® Salsa

Preparation Time: 9 minutes

Cooking Time: 22 minutes

Serving: 12

Size/ Portion: 2 tablespoons

Ingredients:

- 12 cups seeded diced tomatoes
- 6 ounces tomato paste
- 2 medium yellow onions
- 6 small jalapeño peppers
- 4 cloves garlic
- ¼ cup white vinegar
- ¼ cup lime juice
- 2 tablespoons granulated sugar
- 2 teaspoons salt
- ¼ cup chopped fresh cilantro

Direction:

1. Place tomatoes, tomato paste, onions, jalapeños, garlic, vinegar, lime juice, sugar, and salt in the Instant Pot® and stir well. Close it, situate steam release to Sealing. Click Manual button, and time to 20 minutes.

2. Once timer beeps, quick-release the pressure. Open, stir in cilantro, and press the Cancel button.

3. Let salsa cool to room temperature, about 40 minutes, then transfer to a storage container and refrigerate overnight.

Nutrition: 68 Calories 0.1g Fat 2g Protein

Sfougato

Preparation Time: 9 minutes

Cooking Time: 13 minutes

Serving: 4

Size/ Portion: 2 tablespoons

Ingredients:

- ½ cup crumbled feta cheese
- ¼ cup bread crumbs
- 1 medium onion
- 4 tablespoons all-purpose flour
- 2 tablespoons fresh mint
- ½ teaspoon salt
- ½ teaspoon ground black pepper
- 1 tablespoon dried thyme
- 6 large eggs, beaten
- 1 cup water

Direction:

1. In a medium bowl, mix cheese, bread crumbs, onion, flour, mint, salt, pepper, and thyme. Stir in eggs.

2. Spray an 8" round baking dish with nonstick cooking spray. Pour egg mixture into dish.

3. Place rack in the Instant Pot® and add water. Fold a long piece of foil in half lengthwise. Lay foil over rack to form a sling and top with dish. Cover loosely with foil. Seal lid, put steam release in Sealing, select Manual, and time to 8 minutes.

4. When the timer alarms, release the pressure. Uncover. Let stand 5 minutes, then remove dish from pot.

Nutrition: 274 Calories 14g Fat 17g Protein

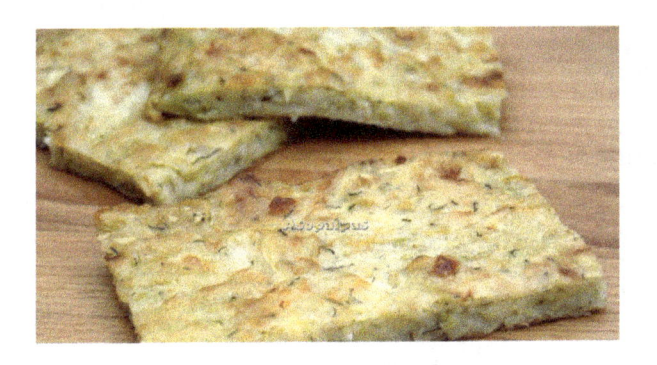

Skordalia

Preparation Time: 7 minutes

Cooking Time: 11 minutes

Serving: 16

Size/ Portion: 2 tablespoons

Ingredients:

- 1-pound russet potatoes
- 3 cups plus ¼ cup water
- 2 teaspoons salt
- 8 cloves garlic
- ¾ cup blanched almonds
- ½ cup extra-virgin olive oil
- 2 tablespoons lemon juice
- 2 tablespoons white wine vinegar
- ½ teaspoon ground black pepper

Direction

1. Place potatoes, 3 cups water, and 1 teaspoon salt in the Instant Pot® and stir well. Close, set steam release to Sealing, click Manual button, and set to 10 minutes.

2. While potatoes cook, place garlic and remaining 1 teaspoon salt on a cutting board. With the side of a knife, press garlic and salt until it forms a paste. Transfer garlic paste into a food processor along with almonds and olive oil. Purée into a paste. Set aside.

3. When the timer beeps, quick-release the pressure. Select Cancel button and open lid. Drain potatoes and transfer to a medium bowl. Add garlic mixture and mash with a potato masher until smooth. Stir in lemon juice, vinegar, and pepper. Stir in ¼ cup water a little at a time until mixture is thin enough for dipping. Serve warm or at room temperature.

Nutrition: 115 Calories 10g Fat 2g Protein

Pinto Bean Dip with Avocado Pico

Preparation Time: 6 minutes

Cooking Time: 52 minutes

Serving: 16

Size/ Portion: 3 tablespoons

Ingredients:

- 1 cup dried pinto beans
- 4 cups water
- 4 tablespoons cilantro, divided
- 3 tablespoons extra-virgin olive oil
- 1 teaspoon ground cumin
- 1 clove garlic, peeled and minced
- ½ teaspoon salt
- 1 medium avocado
- 1 large ripe tomato
- 1 small jalapeño pepper
- ½ medium white onion

- 2 teaspoons lime juice

Direction

1. Place beans, water, and 2 tablespoons cilantro in the Instant Pot®. Close lid, place steam release to Sealing, click Bean and set default time of 30 minutes.

2. When the timer rings, let pressure release naturally. Open then check the beans are tender. Drain off excess water. Crush beans with fork. Add oil, cumin, garlic, and salt and mix well.

3. Toss remaining 2 tablespoons cilantro with avocado, tomato, jalapeño, onion, and lime juice. Spoon topping over bean dip. Serve.

Nutrition: 59 Calories 4g Fat 1g Protein

Power Pods & Hearty Hazelnuts with Mustard-y Mix

Preparation Time: 15 minutes

Cooking Time: 15 minutes

Serving: 4

Size/ Portion: 1-cup

Ingredients:

- 1-lb. green beans, trimmed
- 3-tbsp extra-virgin olive oil (divided)
- 2-tsp whole grain mustard
- 1-tbsp red wine vinegar
- ¼-tsp salt
- ¼-tsp ground pepper
- ¼-cup toasted hazelnuts, chopped

Directions:

1. Preheat your grill to high heat.
2. In a big mixing bowl, toss the green beans with a tablespoon of olive oil. Place the beans in a grill basket.

Grill for 8 minutes until charring a few spots, stirring occasionally.
3. Combine and whisk together the remaining oil, mustard, vinegar, salt, and pepper in the same mixing bowl. Add the grilled beans and toss to coat evenly.
4. To serve, top the side dish with hazelnuts.

Nutrition: 181 Calories 15g Fats 3g Protein

Peppery Potatoes

Preparation Time: 10 minutes

Cooking Time: 18 minutes

Serving: 4

Size/ Portion: 1 cup

Ingredients:

- 4-pcs large potatoes, cubed
- 4-tbsp extra-virgin olive oil (divided)
- 3-tbsp garlic, minced
- ½-cup coriander or cilantro, finely chopped
- 2-tbsp fresh lemon juice
- 1¾-tbsp paprika
- 2-tbsp parsley, minced

Directions:

1. Place the potatoes in a microwave-safe dish. Pour over a tablespoon of olive oil. Cover the dish tightly with plastic wrap. Heat the potatoes for seven minutes in your microwave to par-cook them.

2. Cook 2 tablespoons of olive oil in a pan placed over medium-low heat. Add the garlic and cover. Cook for 3 minutes. Add the coriander, and cook 2 minutes. Transfer the garlic-coriander sauce in a bowl, and set aside.
3. In the same pan placed over medium heat, heat 1 tablespoon of olive oil. Add the par-cooked potatoes. Do not stir! Cook for 3 minutes until browned, flipping once with a spatula. Continue cooking until browning all the sides.
4. Take out the potatoes and place them on a dish. Pour over the garlic-coriander sauce and lemon juice. Add the paprika, parsley, and salt. Toss gently to coat evenly.

Nutrition: 316.2 Calories 14.2g Fats 4.5g Protein

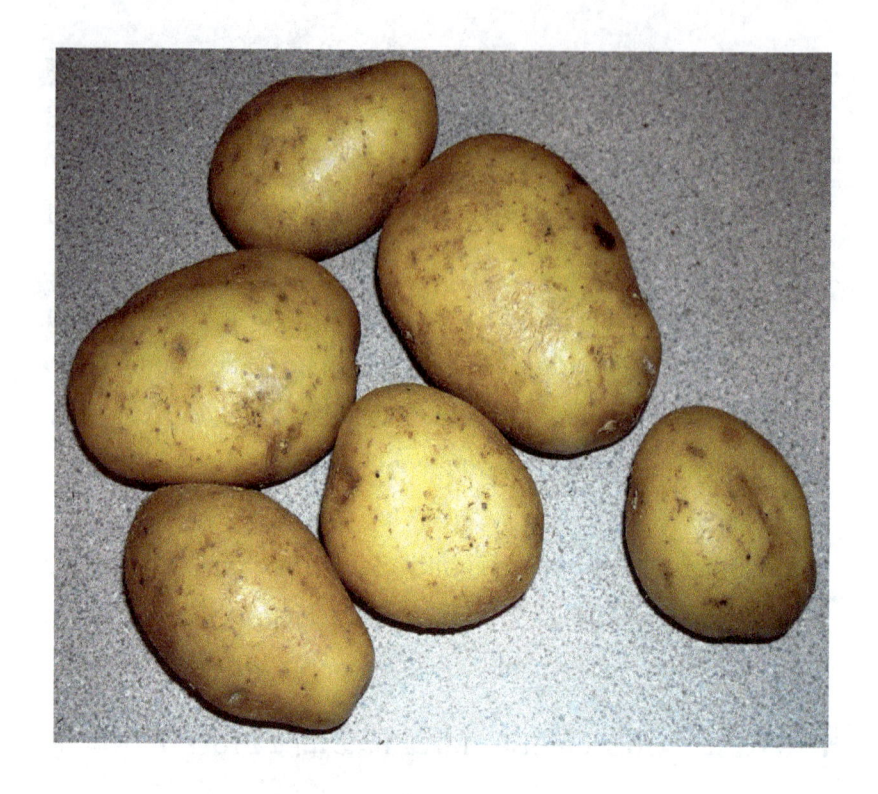

Turkey Spheroids with Tzatziki Sauce

Preparation Time: 10 minutes

Cooking Time: 20 minutes

Serving: 8

Size/ Portion: 2 meatballs

Ingredients:

For Meatballs:

- 2-lbs ground turkey
- 2-tsp salt
- 2-cups zucchini, grated
- 1-tbsp lemon juice
- 1-cup crumbled feta cheese
- 1½-tsp pepper
- 1½-tsp garlic powder
- 1½-tbsp oregano
- ¼-cup red onion, finely minced

For Tzatziki Sauce:

- 1-tsp garlic powder
- 1-tsp dill
- 1-tbsp white vinegar
- 1-tbsp lemon juice
- 1-cup sour cream
- ½-cup grated cucumber
- Salt and pepper

Directions:

1. Preheat your oven to 350 °F.
2. For the Meatballs:
3. Incorporate all the meatball ingredients in a large mixing bowl. Mix well until fully combined. Form the turkey mixture into spheroids, using ¼-cup of the mixture per spheroid.
4. Heat a non-stick skillet placed over high heat. Add the meatballs, and sear for 2 minutes.
5. Transfer the meatballs in a baking sheet. Situate the sheet in the oven, and bake for 15 minutes.
6. For the Tzatziki Sauce:
7. Combine and whisk together all the sauce ingredients in a medium-sized mixing bowl. Mix well until fully

combined. Refrigerate the sauce until ready to serve and eat.

Nutrition: 280 Calories 16g Fats 26.6g Protein

Cheesy Caprese Salad Skewers

Preparation Time: 15 minutes

Cooking Time: 0 minute

Serving: 10

Size/ Portion: 2 skewers

Ingredients:

- 8-oz cherry tomatoes, sliced in half
- A handful of fresh basil leaves, rinsed and drained
- 1-lb fresh mozzarella, cut into bite-sized slices
- Balsamic vinegar
- Extra virgin olive oil
- Freshly ground black pepper

Directions:

1. Sandwich a folded basil leaf and mozzarella cheese between the halves of tomato onto a toothpick.
2. Drizzle with olive oil and balsamic vinegar each skewer. To serve, sprinkle with freshly ground black pepper.

Nutrition: 94 Calories 3.7g Fats 2.1g Protein

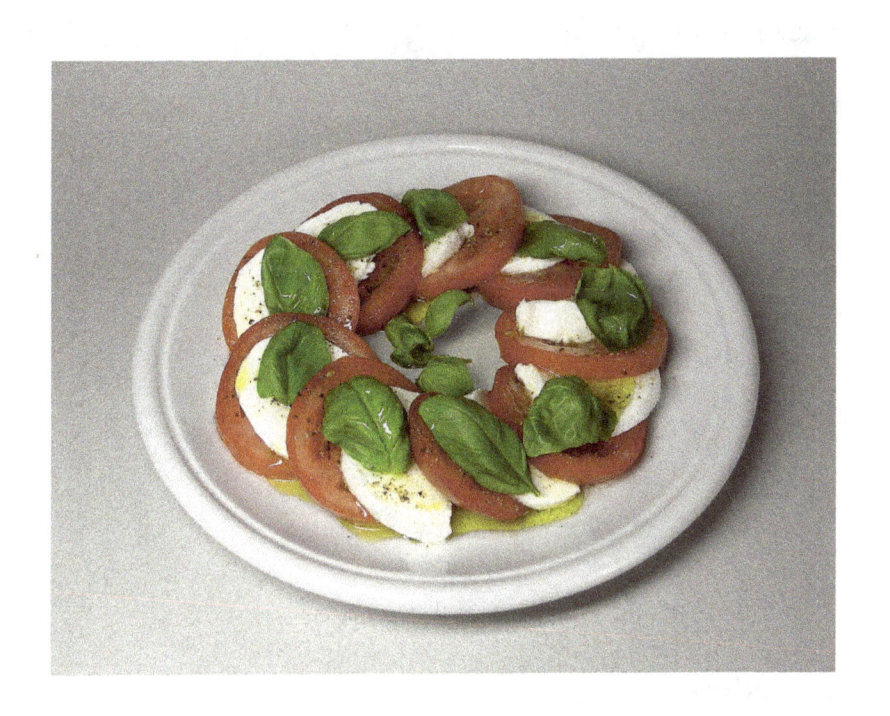

Leafy Lacinato Tuscan Treat

Preparation Time: 10 minutes

Cooking Time: 0 minute

Serving: 1

Size/ Portion: 3 wraps

Ingredients:

- 1-tsp Dijon mustard
- 1-tbsp light mayonnaise
- 3-pcs medium-sized Lacinato kale leaves
- 3-oz. cooked chicken breast, thinly sliced
- 6-bulbs red onion, thinly sliced
- 1-pc apple, cut into 9-slices

Directions:

1. Mix the mustard and mayonnaise until fully combined.
2. Spread the mixture generously on each of the kale leaves. Top each leaf with 1-oz. chicken slices, 3-apple slices, and 2-red onion slices. Roll each kale leaf into a wrap.

Nutrition: 370 Calories 14g Fats 29g Protein

Greek Guacamole Hybrid Hummus

Preparation Time: 10 minutes

Cooking Time: 0 minute

Serving: 1

Size/ Portion: 1-unit

Ingredients:

- 1-15 oz. canned chickpeas
- 1-pc ripe avocado
- ¼-cup tahini paste
- 1-cup fresh cilantro leaves
- ¼-cup lemon juice
- 1-tsp ground cumin
- ¼-cup extra-virgin olive oil
- 1-clove garlic
- ½ tsp salt

Directions:

1. Drain the chickpeas and reserve 2-tablespoons of the liquid. Pour the reserved liquid in your food processor and add in the drained chickpeas.

2. Add the avocado, tahini, cilantro, lemon juice, cumin, oil, garlic, and salt. Puree the mixture into a smooth consistency.

3. Serve with pita chips, veggie chips, or crudités.

Nutrition: 156 Calories 12g Fats 3g Protein

Portable Packed Picnic Pieces

Preparation Time: 5 minutes

Cooking Time: 0 minute

Serving: 1

Size/ Portion: 1-set

Ingredients:

- 1-slice of whole-wheat bread, cut into bite-size pieces
- 10-pcs cherry tomatoes
- ¼-oz. aged cheese, sliced
- 6-pcs oil-cured olives

Directions:

1. Pack each of the ingredients in a portable container to serve you while snacking on the go.

Nutrition: 197 Calories 9g Fats 7g Protein

Perfect Pizza & Pastry

Preparation Time: 35 minutes

Cooking Time: 15 minutes

Serving: 10

Size/ Portion: 2 wedges

Ingredients:

For Pizza Dough:

- 2-tsp honey
- ¼-oz. active dry yeast
- 1¼-cups warm water (about 120 °F)
- 2-tbsp olive oil
- 1-tsp sea salt
- 3-cups whole grain flour + ¼-cup, as needed for rolling

For Pizza Topping:

- 1-cup pesto sauce (refer to Perky Pesto recipe)
- 1-cup artichoke hearts

- 1-cup wilted spinach leaves
- 1-cup sun-dried tomato
- ½-cup Kalamata olives
- 4-oz. feta cheese
- 4-oz. mixed cheese of equal parts low-fat mozzarella, asiago, and provolone

Optional:

- Bell pepper
- Chicken breast, strips
- Fresh basil
- Pine nuts

Directions:

For the Pizza Dough:

1. Preheat your oven to 350 °F.
2. Combine the honey and yeast with the warm water in your food processor with a dough attachment. Blend the mixture until fully combined. Allow the mixture to rest for 5 minutes to ensure the activity of the yeast through the appearance of bubbles on the surface.

3. Pour in the olive oil. Add the salt, and blend for half a minute. Add gradually 3 cups of flour, about half a cup at a time, blending for a couple of minutes between each addition.
4. Let your processor knead the mixture for 10 minutes until smooth and elastic, sprinkling it with flour whenever necessary to prevent the dough from sticking to the processor bowl's surfaces.
5. Take the dough from the bowl. Let it stand for 15 minutes, covered with a moist, warm towel.
6. Using a rolling pin, roll out the dough to a half-inch thickness, dusting it with flour as needed. Poke holes indiscriminately on the dough using a fork to prevent crust bubbling.
7. Place the perforated, rolled dough on a pizza stone or baking sheet. Bake for 5 minutes.

For Pizza Topping:

1. Lightly brush the baked pizza shell with olive oil.
2. Pour over the pesto sauce and spread thoroughly over the pizza shell's surface, leaving out a half-inch space around its edge as the crust.
3. Top the pizza with artichoke hearts, wilted spinach leaves, sun-dried tomatoes, and olives. Cover the top with the cheese.
4. Place the pizza directly on the oven rack. Bake for 10 minutes. Set aside for 5 minutes before slicing.

Nutrition: 242.8 Calories 15g Fats 14g Protein

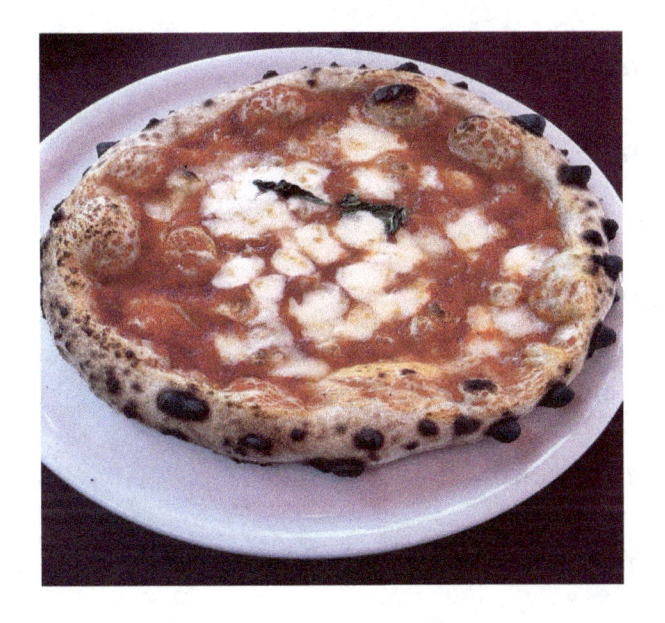

Margherita Mediterranean Model

Preparation Time: 15 minutes

Cooking Time: 15 minutes

Serving: 10

Size/ Portion: 2 wedges

Ingredients:

- 1-batch pizza shell
- 2-tbsp olive oil
- ½-cup crushed tomatoes
- 3-Roma tomatoes, sliced ¼-inch thick
- ½-cup fresh basil leaves, thinly sliced
- 6-oz. block mozzarella
- ½-tsp sea salt

Directions:
1. Preheat your oven to 450 °F.
2. Lightly brush the pizza shell with olive oil. Thoroughly spread the crushed tomatoes over the pizza shell, leaving a half-inch space around its edge as the crust.

3. Top the pizza with the Roma tomato slices, basil leaves, and mozzarella slices. Sprinkle salt over the pizza.
4. Place the pizza directly on the oven rack. Bake for 15 minutes. Put aside for 5 minutes before slicing.

Nutrition: 251 Calories 8g Fats 9g Protein

Fowl & Feta Fettuccini

Preparation Time: 5 minutes

Cooking Time: 30 minutes

Serving: 6

Size/ Portion: 1½-cups

Ingredients:

- 2-tbsp extra-virgin olive oil
- 1½-lb chicken breasts
- ¼-tsp freshly ground black pepper
- 1-tsp kosher salt
- 2-cups water
- 2-14.5-oz. cans tomatoes with garlic, oregano and basil
- 1-lb whole-wheat fettuccini pasta
- 4-oz. reduced-fat feta cheese
- Fresh basil leaves, finely chopped (optional)

Directions:

1. Heat up olive oil for 1 minute in your Dutch oven placed over high heat for 1 minute. Add the chicken, and sprinkle over with freshly ground black pepper and half a teaspoon of kosher salt. Cook the chicken for 8 minutes, flipping once. Sprinkle over with the remaining salt after flipping each chicken on its side. Cook further for 5 minutes until the chicken cooks through.
2. Pour in the water, and add the tomatoes. Stir in the fettuccini pasta, cook for 5 minutes, uncovered. Cover the dish, and cook further for 10 minutes.
3. Uncover the dish, and stir the pasta. Add 3-oz. of the feta cheese, and stir again. Cook further for 5 minutes, uncovered.
4. To serve, sprinkle over with the chopped basil and the remaining feta cheese.

Nutrition: 390 Calories 11g Fats 19g Protein

Very Vegan Patras Pasta

Preparation Time: 5 minutes

Cooking Time: 10 minutes

Serving: 6

Size/ Portion: 1-unit

Ingredients:

- 4-quarts salted water
- 10-oz. gluten-free and whole grain pasta
- 5-cloves garlic, minced
- 1-cup hummus
- Salt and pepper
- 1/3cup water
- ½-cup walnuts
- ½-cup olives
- 2-tbsp dried cranberries (optional)

Directions:

1. Bring the salted water to a boil for cooking the pasta.

2. In the meantime, prepare for the hummus sauce. Combine the garlic, hummus, salt, and pepper with water in a mixing bowl. Add the walnuts, olive, and dried cranberries, if desired. Set aside.
3. Put pasta in the boiling water. Cook the pasta according to the package's specifications. Drain the pasta.
4. Transfer the pasta to a large serving bowl and combine with the sauce.

Nutrition: 329 Calories 12.6g Fats 12g Protein

Scrumptious Shrimp Pappardelle Pasta

Preparation Time: 10 minutes

Cooking Time: 20 minutes

Serving: 4

Size/ Portion: 1½-cup

Ingredients:

- 3-quarts salted water
- 1-lb. jumbo shrimp
- ½-tsp kosher salt
- ¼-tsp black pepper
- 3-tbsp olive oil
- 2-cups zucchini
- 1-cup grape tomatoes
- 1/8 tsp red pepper flakes
- 2-cloves garlic
- 1 tsp zest of 1-pc lemon

- 2-tbsp lemon juice

- 1-tbsp Italian parsley, chopped

- 8-oz. fresh pappardelle pasta

Directions:

1. Bring the salted water to a boil for cooking the pasta.
2. In the meantime, prepare for the shrimp. Combine the shrimp with salt and pepper. Set aside.
3. Heat a tablespoon of oil in a large sauté pan placed over medium heat. Add the zucchini slices and sauté for 4 minutes.
4. Add the grape tomatoes and sauté for 2 minutes. Stir in the salt to combine with the vegetables. Transfer the cooked vegetables to a medium-sized bowl. Set aside.
5. In the same sauté pan, pour in the remaining oil. Switch the heat to medium-low. Add the red pepper flakes and garlic. Cook for 2 minutes.
6. Add the seasoned shrimp, and keep the heat on medium-low. Cook the shrimp for 3 minutes on each side until they turn pinkish.
7. Stir in the zest of lemon and the lemon juice. Mix cooked vegetables back to the pan. Stir to combine with the shrimp. Set aside.
8. Situate pasta in the boiling water. Cook following the manufacturer's specifications until al dente texture. Drain the pasta.

9. Transfer the cooked pasta in a large serving bowl and combine with the lemony-garlic shrimp and vegetables.

Nutrition: 474 Calories 15g Fats 37g Protein

Mixed Mushroom Palermitani Pasta

Preparation Time: 5 minutes

Cooking Time: 30 minutes

Serving: 8

Size/ Portion: 1½-cup

Ingredients:

- 5-quarts salted water
- 3-tbsp olive oil
- 26-oz. assorted wild mushrooms
- 4-cloves garlic, minced
- 1-bulb red onion, diced
- 1-tsp sea salt
- 2-tbsp sherry cooking wine
- 2½-tsp fresh thyme, diced
- 1-lb. linguine pasta
- ¾-cup reserved liquid from cooked pasta
- 6-oz. goat cheese

- ¼-cup hazelnuts

Directions:

1. Bring the salted water to a boil for cooking the pasta.
2. In the meantime, heat the olive oil in a large skillet placed over medium-high heat. Add the mushrooms and sauté for 10 minutes until they brown.
3. Add the garlic, onions, and salt. Sauté for 4 minutes.
4. Stir in the wine, and cook down until the liquid evaporates. Sprinkle with thyme, and set aside.
5. Cook pasta in the boiling water in accordance with the manufacturer's specifications.
6. Before draining the pasta completely, reserve ¾-cup of the pasta liquid.
7. Transfer the cooked pasta in a large serving bowl and combine with the mushroom mixture, pasta liquid, and goat cheese. Toss gently to combine fully until the goat cheese melts completely.
8. To serve, top the pasta with chopped hazelnuts.

Nutrition: 331 Calories 12g Fats 13g Protein

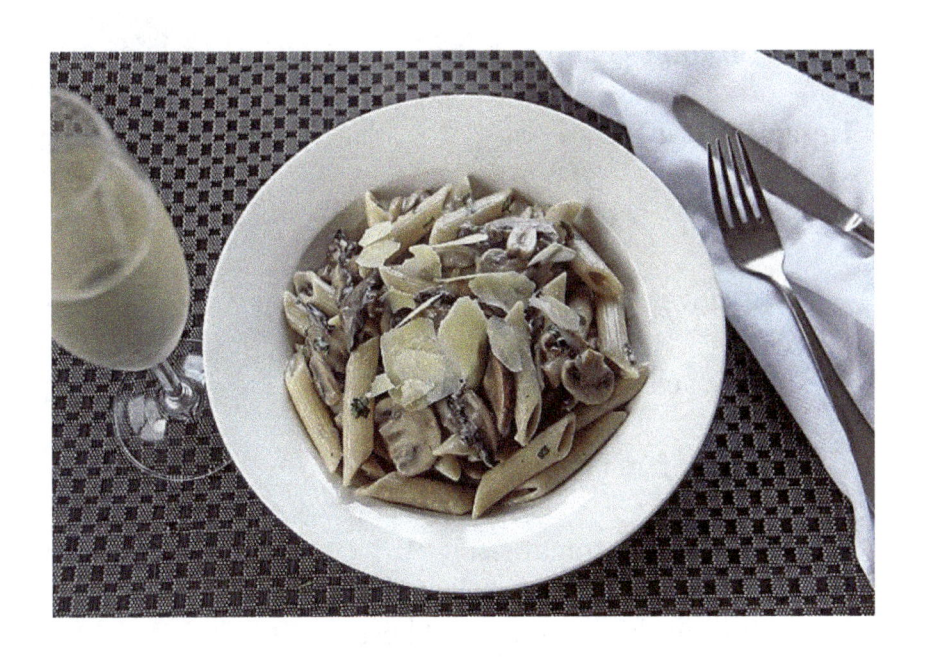

Mediterranean Macaroni with Seasoned Spinach

Preparation Time: 5 minutes

Cooking Time: 20 minutes

Serving: 4

Size/ Portion: 1½-cup

Ingredients:

- 2-tbsp olive oil
- 2-cloves garlic
- 1-pc yellow onion
- 10-oz. fresh baby spinach
- 2-pcs fresh tomatoes
- ¼-cup skim mozzarella cheese
- ½-cup crumbled feta cheese
- ½-cup white cheddar cheese, cubed
- 1-cup low-sodium vegetable broth
- 2-cups elbow whole-grain macaroni

- 1-cup unsweetened almond milk
- ½-tsp organic Italian Seasoning

Directions:

1. Heat up olive oil in a large pan placed over medium-high heat. Add the garlic, onions, and a pinch of salt, and sauté for 3 minutes.
2. Add the spinach, tomatoes, cheese, vegetable broth, macaroni, milk, and seasonings. Mix well until fully combined. Bring the mixture to a boil, stirring frequently.
3. Lower heat to medium-low, and cover the pan. Cook further for 15 minutes, stirring every 3 minutes to prevent the pasta mixture from sticking on the pan's surfaces.
4. Remove the pasta from the heat and stir. To serve, garnish the pasta with parsley.

Nutrition: 544 Calories 23g Fats 22g Protein

Frittata Filled with Zesty Zucchini & Tomato Toppings

Preparation Time: 10 minutes

Cooking Time: 15 minutes

Serving: 4

Size/ Portion: 1-wedge

Ingredients:

- 8-pcs eggs
- ¼-tsp red pepper, crushed
- ¼-tsp salt
- 1-tbsp olive oil
- 1-pc small zucchini
- ½-cup red or yellow cherry tomatoes
- 1/3-cup walnuts, coarsely chopped
- 2-oz. bite-sized fresh mozzarella balls (bocconcini)

Directions:

1. Preheat your broiler. Meanwhile, whisk together the eggs, crushed red pepper, and salt in a medium-sized bowl. Set aside.
2. In a 10-inch broiler-proof skillet placed over medium-high heat, heat the olive oil. Arrange the slices of zucchini in an even layer on the bottom of the skillet. Cook for 3 minutes, turning them once, halfway through.
3. Top the zucchini layer with cherry tomatoes. Pour the egg mixture over vegetables in skillet. Top with walnuts and mozzarella balls.
4. Switch to medium heat. Cook for 5 minutes. By using a spatula, lift the frittata for the uncooked portions of the egg mixture to flow underneath.
5. Place the skillet on the broiler. Broil the frittata 4-inches from the heat for 5 minutes until the top is set. To serve, cut the frittata into wedges.

Nutrition: 281 Calories 14g Fats 17g Protein

Conclusion

The Mediterranean diet considers various aspects of what "health" means. It does not just focus on what you eat but it also focuses on how you eat, who you eat with, and the activities you do in between eating. Each of these components can contribute to better health and a more fulfilling life. When we are lacking in any of these components, we tend to suffer from poor health, fatigue, depression and more. The Mediterranean diet was originally looked at because of its heart health benefits, but now it is clear to see that the traditional Mediterranean lifestyle from the 1950s was more than just a heart-healthy plan.

This book has helped you understand not only the benefits of this diet but has revealed effective tips and suggestions to help you transition into this type of diet. The changes can be made in small steps, because even the smallest change to shifting your diet to a more Mediterranean diet can have a whirlwind of benefits. You have learned how to swap the unhealthy foods you have been used to consuming with nutrient-dense and wholesome foods.

The Mediterranean diet is more than what you eat; it is a way of living. This diet reflects the true definition of what a diet should be. It encourages eating healthy nutritious foods, while also emphasizing the importance of physical activity and spending time with those we care about. The Mediterranean diet has been studied for decades and each time it seems a new benefit of this diet comes to light.

What needs to be done is adopting a new way of looking at food and mealtimes. Our world today stresses working harder and longer which means there is little time for enjoying meals. If we can change our perspective to see that the food, we eat is what makes us more efficient and productive, then we would be able to more easily change the way we eat.

This book has introduced you to what the Mediterranean diet is. It has helped you understand that this isn't your typical diet. That instead, the Mediterranean diet is about changing into a lifestyle that will bring you better health and happiness. This book has provided you with some of the findings from scientific research that supports the diet's benefits. You have learned that the diet consists of eating plenty of fresh fruits, vegetables, and healthy fats like extra virgin olive oil. You still have the freedom to indulge with brain-boosting fish, heart-healthy whole grains, and seafood and sporadically can enjoy a nice steak dinner. This diet is not limiting you to be mindful of your calorie intake or not to consume other important food groups.

The recipes in this book allow you to begin trying out delicious, flavorful, and healthy Mediterranean inspired meals. You have a number of breakfasts, lunch, and dinner options that are sure to satisfy and please everyone in your home. These recipes can be your starting point in taking control of your health.

You now have a better understanding that this diet is not about just losing weight. It is not a diet that allows you to eat your weight in pasta, or drink equal amounts of red wine. It has shown that you can use food as a form of natural medicine to reduce and eliminate the risk of many serious health conditions. You have learned how your food directly affects the way your body functions and when it is deprived of the nutrients it needs it will not be able to perform appropriately.

Now that you have all this information on how you can maintain and achieve optimal health, it is up to you to decide. Will you continue to choose a life where the foods you eat leads you down a road to illness and preventable suffering? Or will you make the change now to live your life and be the healthiest and happiest version of you? All you have to do is start with one small change and then go from there. Once you begin to see the benefits from that one small choice you will be eager to try more and soon you will be living a Mediterranean lifestyle that is significantly more satisfying.

Finally, this book was intended to assist you recognize that diet does not need to make you give up some of your beloved foods. Instead, it allows you to find new favorites that will improve your overall health. Allow the food you enjoy today to be your medicine for your future.